Executive Wellness

The 4 Week
Get-Back-On-Track Program

By

Sam Hester

Houston, Texas

Contents:

"Winning is a habit.
Watch your thoughts,
they become your beliefs.
Watch your beliefs,
they become your words.
Watch your words,
they become your actions.
Watch your actions,
they become your habits.
Watch your habits,
they become your character."

Vince Lombardi

Introduction

This book is designed for busy executives who, by the very nature of their profession, work incredibly long hours, remain sedentary for long stints, are under constant stress, and often have to travel for business. If that describes you, then you may have gotten off track in taking care of your most precious natural asset—**you**!

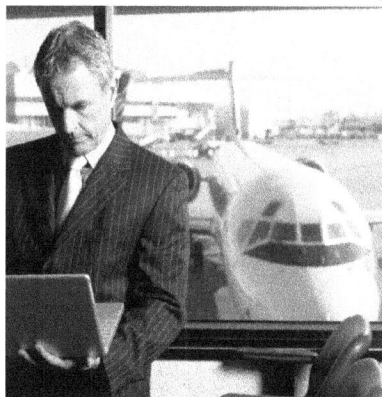

One of the natural consequences of working this much—and having too little free time to pursue your own wellness—is that you reach for food that may be convenient, but is not necessarily healthy for you. Most of it is probably filled with sugar, and so sets a pattern in which about every 2-4 hours, your blood sugar will drop and your body will signal to you that it needs energy. When this vicious cycle emerges, it is often very difficult to break. Another consequence to this cycle is that you don't have the energy to exercise, so you continue to sit and eat and can't get out of the rut!

If that describes your life right now, then I can help. This book is designed to assist you in getting out of the ditch and guide you along the first part of your journey back to better health and wellbeing. I have designed a 4-week program called Get-Back-On-Track (GBOT) that will eliminate your sugar cravings and help you to regain your focus and energy, maximize your productivity, remain resilient, and begin exercising.

My intention in writing this book was based upon my experience at looking how our bodies are made—how our physiology works—and how far away from that we have gotten in our current lifestyles. In my earlier book, *Soar to Success—Minus the Stress* (ISBN: 978-0-615-23238-6), I described how stress is affecting all of us and even killing a number of us, because we don't understand how our bodies function and how our lives today are way out of sync with how we are made.

There are certain laws of life—cause and effect—that should not be violated, and there is a price to be paid when we do. It's not our modern world that's the problem; it's the fact that our bodies have functioned in a certain way for thousands of years, and the more our modern behavior is *misaligned* with that natural functioning, the more problems we end up having.

When you are young, it's possible to be fit but not necessarily *healthy*. However, with rare exceptions, when you're over 40, you have to be *healthy* to be fit. This is a crucial distinction. So, if you focus on getting healthy *first*, then you can become fit and lose weight *much more easily*.

Genetics plays, at most, about 30% in determining your future, and that the other 70% is a product of our lifestyle choices. This reminds me of the line from *Invictus*, by the British poet Henley: "I am the master of my fate, I am the captain of my soul." The good news is that we know a lot more about how to take care of ourselves than ever before in history—even more than we did 10 years ago!

On February 24, 2000, several of the nation's best-known diet gurus, including Dr. Robert Atkins and Dr. Dean Ornish, participated in the USDA's "Great Nutrition Debate," where they discussed their diametrically-opposed ideas about eating, nutrition, and health. Drs. Atkins and Ornish did agree on two things that summed up the essence of the problem: *we eat too much simple sugar, and we don't exercise enough.*

Shazam! That information has stuck with me since then, and building on my interest in the physiological aspects of stress and my coaching hundreds of clients,

I have some insights to share with those of you who are struggling with weight loss, have sugar cravings, and find it difficult to begin exercising again. I do not claim to have "the answer," but I do believe that my gift is taking all of this great body of information and distilling it down into some essentials that people can understand and incorporate in their busy lives. It's like those fundamentals in football: blocking and tackling. If you don't do those things right first, you won't end up winning many games.

Change

Many of us have thought that change was an event, such as *I am quitting smoking today*, or *I am beginning a diet*, which often gets mixed results—the proverbial one step forward, two steps back. Through research, we now know that the *trans-theoretical model* necessary to institute change in our lives is a process, not an event, and that we generally don't begin to make changes until we experience significant discomfort in our continued lifestyle behaviors.

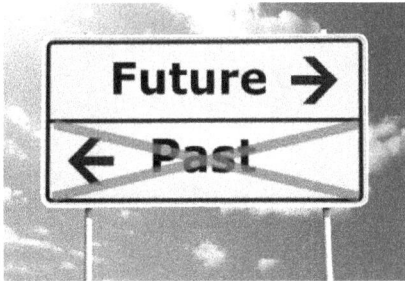

Much like the famed five-staged grief process that Dr. Elizabeth Kübler-Ross introduced in the 1960s, psychologists have identified five different stages that people either consciously or unconsciously pass through on their way to making changes in their lives.

The pattern (see diagram on page 10) is circular (global vs. linear thinking) and that one phase doesn't necessarily involve a conscious thought process.

For example, you keep seeing TV commercials exhorting you to join a gym for $0 down and $29 per month. At first you might think, *Gee that's nice, but I'm not ready to do anything now* (pre-contemplation stage). Several months later, you see the same commercial, and you think, *That seems like a good idea, and I think I'll check that out sometime soon* (contemplation stage).

A couple of weeks go by and then you see the same commercial, and this time you jot down the 800 number and web address and leave it handy on the counter so that it will serve as a reminder (preparation stage). A few more weeks go by, and as you are dressing in the morning, the new suit you bought and haven't worn yet doesn't fit, and in your mind you say, *All right, I am going to call the gym today and get a free two-week membership.* And later in the day, you call and arrange the free trial membership. At this point, you have taken a step and actually done something (action stage). Voila! This is the psychological juncture where all positive change takes place.

You actually show up at the gym, take advantage of the free two-week membership, and begin doing some exercise—and feel good about it. Somewhere in the next several weeks, you will come to a decision point: to continue taking positive steps, such as signing up for some personal training, or to stop going to the gym and slide back into your old ways. It is only through repetition that good habits are developed. Then, continued positive habits lead to success. The objective is to continue taking positive

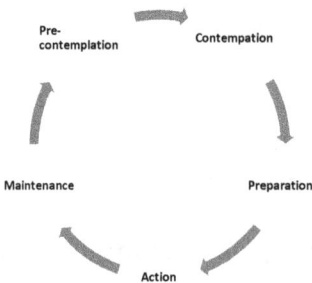

actions until this becomes second nature, and you start feeling results (maintenance stage).

Having seen hundreds of people go through this process, my job is to meet them where they're at (they usually don't call until they are at the action stage) and to help motivate them until they can see and feel some real success from their own perspective. It is very rewarding to see people "get it."

Even a little change is good

Let's use an analogy about the time value of money. How does an initial investment of $1,000 become $10,000? The answer is compound interest. Every time interest is applied, it's not just to the initial $1,000, but also to the current balance, and so forth. Interest over time! How does this idea work in regard to our health and wellness?

Let's say that you eat one fewer cookie a day, and make no other changes in your life. Eating 100 fewer calories per day yields a calorie deficit of 36,500 per year, and since there are 3,500 calories per pound, you will lose a little more than 10 pounds over the course of a year. If you can begin looking at change in this way, it can be highly motivating and exciting.

Wellness vs. diet & fitness

One of the differences in the new paradigm of looking at nutrition, fitness, and weight loss together instead of separately is the new holistic concept of *wellness*: if you start taking action in one part, it will inevitably and positively influence the rest. Let's take a concrete example. You go into your garage and get out the old mountain bike that you haven't ridden since last fall, you put a little oil on one part of the chain, and you begin turning the pedal. The oil begins to lubricate not only that part of the chain, but also other parts of the chain and the gears, as well. So, a little investment in putting some oil on a small part of the chain yields a greater benefit than just the initial action.

In just the same way, if you become more aware of what you eat, and make better choices more of the time, you will overcome your sugar cravings, which will give you more energy to begin exercising, as well. Let's get started!

Food

Infrequent food supply

The human body has not substantially changed since we humans broke off from the Neanderthals over 30,000 years ago. Our forefathers roamed always in search of food, and their bodies had to go without eating for long periods of time. When the kill was made, they gorged themselves to get through until the next meal. Their bodies adapted to work this way to meet the harsh conditions.

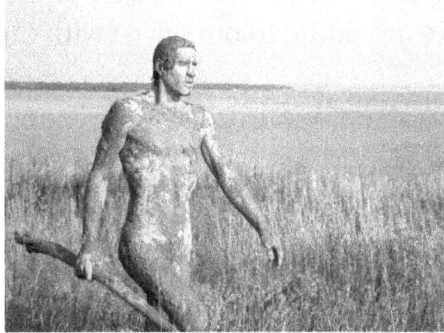

As a result of these adaptations, our hormonal metabolism developed extraordinary *feasting* and *fasting* survival mechanisms so that we could store fat for those periods of time when there was little or nothing to eat. The one constant was early man's level of physical activity, whether he had something to eat or not. Walking 20 or 30 miles was the day's agenda. *We cannot interpret our body's natural needs outside this context.*

Our new normal, for most of us, at least, is a constant and inexhaustible food supply that is available with little or no effort required on our part to obtain it. Imagine if you went out to your car in the morning, turned it on, and let it idle for about 10 minutes, and then turned the car off and tried to put gas into an already-full tank. In our cars, the extra gas would simply overflow, and spill out onto the ground, but our bodies store extra calories not needed at the time as *fat*. Using this analogy, you can begin to see what we are doing to ourselves with our modern lifestyle.

Information is the key

It is shocking, considering all of our current understanding of nutrition and human physiology, how many highly-educated professionals have no clue as to what they are eating and how it affects not only their waistlines, but how they feel and how productive they will be throughout the day.

One of my clients, a terrifically successful investment banker and Wharton Business School Graduate in his fifties, had never read anything about nutrition and didn't have a clue about what he was eating. He just knew that the corn flakes in his pantry were *supposed* to be good for him because it said so on the box. In about 30 minutes, I imparted to him some clear and easy-to-understand information that he was able to utilize immediately and that helped him to control his sugar cravings and improve his productivity *that same day*.

Most people get hungry about every 2-4 hours, as their blood sugar begins to drop. By incorporating some suggestions, within a matter of about a week you will notice that you no longer crave sugary foods, you rarely get hungry, you have more energy to exercise, and you can avoid that afternoon slump that you thought was normal.

Food as fuel

As I jokingly say, I teach people to start thinking about food as molecules. It isn't very sexy, but it shifts the thinking away from surface conversations about food such as "Oh, doesn't that dessert taste good," or "Did you get that new recipe?" to an understanding about what happens after it leaves your fork and enters your body.

Until you can make the connection that food is primarily fuel for your body and that you have it within your power to control your fuel supply, you will continue to muddle along without taking charge of your life, and think you are at the mercy of fate. There is a long-standing saying in some self-help programs that goes "If you keep doing what you have always done, you will continue to get what you have always gotten."

To succeed in the new paradigm, you will not have to go out and spend a lot of money on strange and exotic foods, but rather to utilize your current stores in different ways. All that I ask is that you keep an open mind, and if you want different results than you've gotten in the past, try my suggestions. They are simple, easy, and best of all, they work!

Grease, caffeine, sugar, and chocolate

During the annual Houston Livestock Show and Rodeo, I sometimes tell out-of-town visitors that these are the local four basic food groups. But seriously, everything that you put in your mouth can be classified as protein, carbohydrates, fat, fiber, or water. We will examine each of these elements one at a time.

Read the damn labels!

If the majority of the food that you buy comes from a grocery store, the good news is that there is a label called **Nutrition Facts** that by law has to be on all food products sold in the U.S. This is a very crowded label that has a lot of useful but confusing information that is beyond the scope of our current focus of getting you back-on-track.

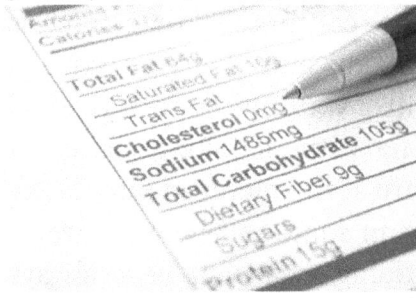

I suggest that you get into the habit of reading labels. But for our purposes, just read these 3 elements:

- Serving size/weight
- Calories per serving
- Total amounts of fat, carbohydrates, and protein

It's not about the weight—really!

Most people begin any meaningful conversation about eating, nutrition, or weight loss by first telling me how much they weigh. When I tell them I don't care what their weight is, I sometimes get some astonished looks. *It's about the fat, not the weight.* Luckily, we have some pretty accurate techniques that will provide us specific information other than our weight.

Lean body mass and body fat percentage

The part of your body that we actually want to feed is called your Lean Body Mass (LBM) or fat-free mass, which is all of the bones, tissue, blood, organs, water, etc., in your body. This is everything but adipose tissue (fat). The LBM is measured in pounds, and is the numerical reciprocal of the more commonly known term–Body Fat Percentage (BF%). The important thing to know about this is that *we don't need to feed the fat.*

> Example: Fred, a sedentary 200-pound corporate executive, has an LBM of 150 pounds. This would mean that he has 50 pounds of fat in his body and his Body Fat Percentage (BF%) is 25 percent – which is the numerical reciprocal of his LBM (200 x 0.25 = 150). So, instead of his scale weight of 200 pounds, I would focus on the 150 pounds, which is the part of the body that we want to nourish and feed.

If you calculate LBM correctly, then you know what your BF% is and vice versa. There are several different ways to accurately estimate these numbers. Among these are:

- Jackson & Pollock body caliper method
- Hydrostatic Underwater method
- Hip-to-waist ratio method
- Bioelectric Impedance Analysis (BIA) method

My personal favorite in working with clients is the Bioelectric Impedance Analysis (BIA), which is a scale-like device you stand on that runs a current through your body (you can't feel it). Based on your gender, height, age, activity level, and the amount of resistance that the signal receives, it can calculate this number very accurately using pre-determined algorithms.

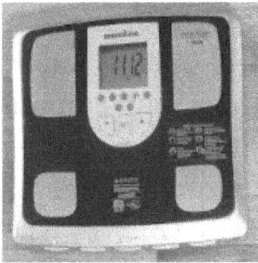

Your local gym or personal trainer probably has access to this technology. I suggest that you seek professional guidance in accurately assessing your LBM/BF. But, since many of you will not have immediate access to one of the methods to determine your LBM, let's approximate the amount of body fat you have and get started. It will get us where we need to go.

Approximate body fat%

If you look naked into a full-length mirror and you don't have any love handles and your stomach is pretty flat, you have about 15% BF if you are a man and about 22%BF if you are a woman. These are optimal BF% for adults.

If you are about average, with small love handles but no rollover gut, then use 22%BF if you are a man and 32%BF if you are a woman.

If you are about 10-20% above your ideal weight (most adults in the U.S.), then if you are a man you are at about 30%BF and a woman, about 40%BF.

If you are 30% or higher above your ideal weight, use 37%BF if you are a man, and 45%BF if you are a woman. If you are heavier than this, then use these numbers anyway, which will still serve you to get you started.

Calculating your lean body mass

_____Actual Weight in Pounds

- _____Total Body Fat in Pounds

(Actual Weight x BF%
converted to pounds)

= _____Lean Body Mass (LBM)

Use food like a drug

You may have heard the old saying by Hippocrates, considered the Father of Medicine, "Let your food be your medicine, and let your medicine be your food." You might think this is merely a quaint old proverb, but you will learn that you can control your sugar cravings with food, much like your doctor gives you a medication to control a certain health problem. He or she understands the half-life of the drug and directs you in the prescription as to how much and how often you should take it to keep it stable in your bloodstream in order to gain the maximum targeted effect in treating your medical condition.

We are going to do the same thing with certain foods, especially protein. To sum up the process, it's not only what we eat, but how much we eat, when we eat it, and how often. This is my proverb!

Protein

Much like concrete and steel are the foundations of building structures, proteins make up the building blocks of our organs, body parts, and enzymes, and do all of the maintenance and repair functions as well. Proteins are made up of 20 different amino acids, of which the body by itself manufactures 11. The other 9 are called "essential amino acids," meaning that the

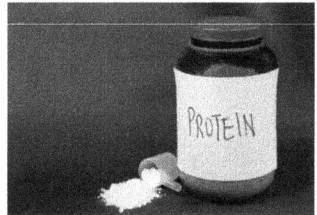

body cannot produce them; they must come from some outside food source.

All animal and dairy-based protein food sources are considered "complete" proteins. This means they contain all 20 of the amino acids required by the body. Other plant-based sources, such as beans and legumes, have some but not all of the 20 amino acids. That's why vegetarians must combine different sources to make sure that they get all of their needed complete protein. All protein sources have 4 calories per gram.

The magic of protein

Protein is the most potent weapon that you can use to help control your hormonal balances and, more importantly, keep your blood sugar stable. Anytime that you eat protein it triggers the release of **Glucagon,** the fasting hormone, from your pancreas. It actually raises your blood sugar levels and also signals the body to release the glycogen (sugar) stores in your liver and to mobilize your body to begin burning fat for fuel.

Protein Prescription (PP)

So how much protein do you need to feed and support your LBM? To calculate your daily protein needs, or what it is commonly called your Protein Prescription (PP), you need to determine the routine activity level that you engage in on an average day. Choose the most appropriate level below.

Physical Activity Level Per Average Day	Grams of Protein per pound of LBM
Sedentary: no real exercise or activity except activities of daily living	0.6
Modestly Active: light yard work, housecleaning, running errands	0.7
Moderately Active: leisurely walking, golfing, strenuous yard work	0.8
Active Lifestyle: walk/run/cycle at least 3x week for 30 min.	0.9
Very Active: run/cycle/swim 5x week for 60 min.	1.0

Your LBM is _____ X _____ Grams of Protein per Pound/LBM = _____ Total Grams of Protein Per Day (TGPD).

Example:

Sarah is a 55-year-old national sales manager whose LBM is 107 pounds x 0.8 (moderately active) = 85.6 TGPD. Rounding slightly up, she should eat approximately 90 TGPD. (Always round up, as it's better to get a little too much protein than too little.)

Divide 90 by 5 = 18 grams of protein that Sarah needs to consume at every meal. This is called her Total Grams of Protein Per Meal (TGPM).

Your TGPD = _____ and then divide that number by 5 = _____ Total Grams of Protein Per Meal (TGPM).

Breakfast   _____TGPM
Morning Snack   _____TGPM
Lunch   _____TGPM
Afternoon Snack _____TGPM
Dinner   _____TGPM

The closer that you can keep to this 3-hour rule—especially at first, until you see how your body reacts—the better your results will be. Remember I said earlier that about every 2-4 hours most peoples' blood sugar begins to drop, so we are using protein to help keep your blood sugar stable.

The body can only digest and utilize at most about 30-35 grams of protein at any one time. If you eat more than that, the liver automatically converts the leftover protein into fat. *So never eat more than 35 grams of protein at any one setting. Remember, it's not only what you eat, but how much and how often, that makes the difference.*

Sources of protein

The good news is that you don't have to eat just meat to get your TGPM. You can eat a variety of vegetables, nuts, dairy, or my favorites, soy or whey protein powders.

Whey is a milk-based product and is a great source of easily digestible protein, unless you have dietary or health issues around the consumption of dairy products. Soy is the only plant-based food that is a complete protein, and is another great choice in obtaining your daily protein. I have seen amazing results from people using protein powders, either mixed in a shaker, made into a smoothie, or any other creative way that you can think of to utilize the powders.

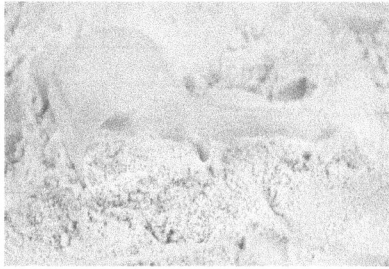

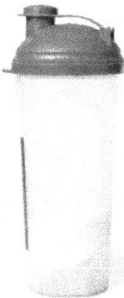

You can put it in a small baggie and label it Protein Powder, and it fits nicely into your briefcase or carry-on luggage along with your shaker. Mix it with water and you are good for the next 3 hours. The TSA is pretty good about understanding this, especially if you put it out with your belt and shoes and they can see the label. I have never heard of anyone having a problem with this.

You can find whey and soy powders in any grocery or health food store as well as Sam's Club and Costco. Whey comes from a number of different sources, so I would encourage you to buy the least expensive option, as long as it states 100% whey, and try it first. The vanilla flavor is the easiest to mix; even with water, the taste is pretty good. If you are lactose intolerant, you might try Whey Protein Isolate (WPI), as it has little or no lactose in it.

There are many other sources of good information for you to get ideas to meet your optimal protein requirements. Pay attention to the labels and get your TGPM.

Carbohydrates

If you ask someone what type of food an apple or broccoli is, they will generally answer a fruit or a vegetable. Interestingly, most people don't know that they are both carbohydrates ("carbs").

Fruits, vegetables, starches (e.g., potatoes, rice, pasta, grains, bread, etc.) and dairy products contain mostly carbohydrates, which when broken down in the body, all turn into sugar. *All carbohydrates are sugar.*

Once you eat foods that contain carbs, they are digested and inside the body at the molecular level, converted into **glucose,** which is the scientific term for blood sugar, and is used for fuel for our brain, muscles, and all of the cells in our body.

There has been a lot of misinformation in the media the last few years, either extolling the virtues of carbs as the best thing since sliced bread (pun intended) or the source of all of our weight and health issues. We could not live without carbohydrates for very long. They are neither good nor bad, just a necessary part of the overall food choices that we have available. All carbohydrates have 4 calories per gram, the same number as protein.

What is sugar?

Without getting into a long discussion of carbohydrate metabolism, there are 3 different forms of simple sugars that all carbs are broken down into before the body can utilize them. They are called monosaccharides: glucose, fructose, and galactose. Glucose is primarily in starches and vegetables, fructose is in fruit, and galactose is in dairy products.

What we call *table sugar* is actually one molecule of glucose + one molecule of fructose, which produces a disaccharide called sucrose. This is the correct term for what we call "added sugar," present in many sweets such as desserts and sodas, and what gives them such a good taste. During digestion and food assimilation, the body has to break the sucrose into its two different molecules, glucose and fructose, to be utilized.

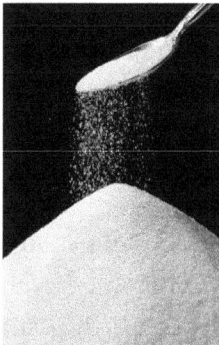

What goes up must come down

Anytime you eat any carbohydrate (sugar), your body secretes **insulin,** the feasting hormone, from your pancreas (remember that **glucagon** was the fasting hormone). Insulin is designed to keep your blood sugar from rising too high and to keep it within a certain narrow, specific range. Insulin plays another very important role that most people do not recognize: it acts like a key and helps unlock the individual cells so that glucose can get inside and be used for energy production.

Nature also assumed that you were going to be on the move most of the time, there would be a constant demand for energy, insulin levels would be maintained at a low level, and everything would work efficiently as designed.

Due to our sedentary lifestyles coupled with eating carbs much of the time; the body has an overabundance of glucose that isn't needed in our cells, so it backs up in our blood. The liver can store a small amount of glucose (about equivalent to 3 candy bars) in the form of glycogen (stored glucose), and when that is full, *the body stores the excess glucose as fat.*

Much has been written in the last decade concerning the deleterious effects of too much insulin floating around the body, including Type 2 diabetes, obesity, heart disease, and cancer. Therefore I will not plow the ground with which many of you already are familiar. Please do check with your doctor about any specific questions that you have on this matter.

Glycemic Index

In addition to getting more exercise to help the insulin unlock the cells so that they can get the needed glucose, we can use our carbohydrate choices to minimize over-production of insulin by the body and maintain a good range of blood sugar values. In the past, most carbs were listed as either simple or complex, with the notion that simple carbs and "sugar'" were the worst choices. Well that information turned out to be wrong.

In 1981, a group of researchers at the University of Toronto asked a better question: How fast do individual carbohydrates actually enter the bloodstream? The result is something called the **Glycemic Index**. It actually measures the rate of release into the bloodstream relative to pure glucose, which has an assigned value of 100. The scale goes from 0 to 100 and lists almost every food available. There are a few foods that have a value over 100. The lower the Glycemic Index (GI) value, the slower the rate of release of glucose into the bloodstream and more importantly, the less insulin produced.

The value can be affected by the amount of protein, fat, or fiber in the food itself, and especially the fat, which can act as a brake to help slow down the absorption rate.

Below is a working list of the Glycemic Index for some popular foods, in no particular order.

High Glycemic Index	GI Value	Moderate Glycemic Index	GI Value	Low Glycemic Index	GI Value
70 & above		55 - 69		54 or less	
Cornflakes Cereal	81	New Potato	57	Soy Milk	30
White Bread	71	Oat Bran Cereal	55	Apple Juice	41
Rice Krispies Cereal	82	Brown Rice	55	All Bran Cereal	42
White Rice	73	Whole Wheat Bread	69	Fruit Yogurt	41
Potato, instant/Mashed	87	Popcorn	55	Regular Milk	39
Waffles	76	Raisins	64	Asparagus	15
Doughnut	76	Spaghetti, durum wheat	55	Lettuce	15
Corn Chips	74	Green Banana	55	Ice Cream	51
Pretzels	81	French Fries	63	Almonds	15
Jelly Beans	80	Danish Pastry	59	Soybeans	16
Gatorade	78	Soft Drink/Soda	59	Spinach	15

For a complete list of the GI value of any food, go to **www.glycemicindex.com**. When I refer to low GI, it means a carb choice with a GI value **under 55**.

For breakfast, lunch, and dinner, I would suggest that you concentrate on choosing **low GI starches and vegetables**, and eating these food groups together.

They all utilize glucose directly, and should be eaten **separately from fruits and dairy products**.

Eat fruits and dairy products together

For your morning and afternoon snack, along with your protein I suggest that you eat either fruit or milk-based carbs such as yogurt or cheese. You can eat either one or both together but **separate from vegetables and starches**.

They have low GI values and here's why. The primary monosaccharide (simple) sugar in fruit (fructose) and milk (galactose) both have to be converted into glucose by going through the liver, which can take up to 20 minutes, since the body doesn't have the enzymes to utilize fructose and galactose directly as it does glucose.

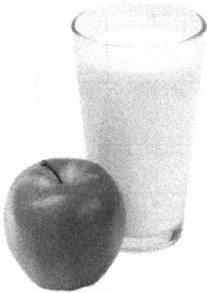

Consequently, you only want to eat small quantities of these at any one time, since the liver can only store a small amount of glycogen at any one time. If you eat fructose and/or galactose by themselves and separate from the starches and vegetables, you have a very limited insulin response and it will automatically help keep your blood sugar stable. So, eating small amounts of fruits and dairy products with protein snacks is a perfect opportunity.

Fats

There has been much written over the last decade about the "good and bad fats" and the different types of oils, so again, I will not say much here of a general nature. All food sources of fat have 9 calories per gram, while carbs and protein have only 4 calories per gram.

Eating fat does not make you fat

Let's face it, foods high in fat taste good and give us a feeling of satiety (feeling full). That's the main reason that we eat them in abundance. Our bodies actually need fats; in fact, we could not live without them. They are a source of energizing fuel, help keep our skin soft, are fundamental in assisting with essential fatty acids, and help to deliver fat-soluble vitamins. And, even more importantly for your waistline, *fat does not evoke an insulin response and can assist in slowing down the rate of release of sugar into the bloodstream when eaten with carbs.*

Nuts

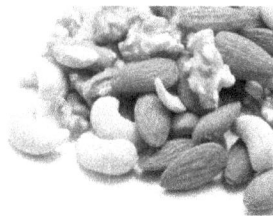

Most of the nuts and seeds are not only very good choices to get your "good fats," but they are also inexpensive and easily transported. Cashews, hazelnuts, and almonds are packed full of monounsaturated fats, and walnuts are very rich in omega-3 fats. The trick is to eat just a few at a time. For example, a handful of 20-25 almonds (approximately one ounce) have approximately 160 nutrient-rich calories.

Read the labels so that you are aware of nuts' overall calorie count. I highly recommend that you eat nuts with your morning and afternoon snacks. Most of my clients find them an excellent source of needed "good fats." Also, like your protein powder, nuts travel very well.

Fiber

Most of what we hear from doctors and health experts is that we all need more fiber. But what is dietary fiber? It used to be called "roughage" and we vaguely know that it has something to do with digestion and maintaining good bowel habits. It is mostly found in fruits, vegetables, legumes, whole grains, seeds, and nuts. There are two types of fiber: soluble and insoluble. As the names suggest, soluble fiber dissolves in water and insoluble fiber does not.

Soluble fiber acts like a sponge and attracts water, and it also aids in slowing down digestion, which can make you feel full and lower the glycemic index in the food.

On the other hand, insoluble fiber does not dissolve in water, and passes through the intestinal tract easily without breaking down much; it assists other foods in passing the gut. Insoluble fiber has a laxative effect, enabling elimination and helping to prevent constipation.

If a client asks me how much fiber they should eat, my general suggestion is simple: more! As has been said, one of the benefits of eating more fruits and vegetables is "staying regular." You will know when you are eating too much roughage and need to cut back a bit.

Water

The human body is about 60 percent water. The blood is composed of about 92 percent water; the muscles and brain are about 75 percent, and bones are about 22 percent. So obtaining sufficient daily water intake is obviously an important thing to achieve.

In the media, we are again told that we should drink x number of glasses or y ounces of water daily. And, so the unspoken assumption is that if we don't do *exactly* that, then we are not keeping ourselves properly hydrated. For most busy people, they are not going to follow this admonition, so I want to give you a different way of looking at this.

Cow's milk is about 87 percent water; fruits and vegetables are generally between about 80 to 95 percent water and even decaffeinated sugar-free diet sodas/teas etc. are about 99 percent water. Even after you take into account the diuretic effect of caffeinated drinks such as diet sodas, coffee and tea, it is estimated that your body is still getting about two thirds of the liquid as water.

Yes, the human body was meant to drink only milk and water–but by eating more fruits and vegetables along with drinking more of the other more palatable everyday drinks–your body still should be able to get the daily amount of water it needs. If a client asks me how much water (liquid) they should drink, my suggestion is again simple: more. If you are thirsty, your body is already becoming dehydrated, so drink up!

Calculating Calories

There is still a lot of debate among nutrition and medical experts about the role of counting calories as a part of an overall health, nutrition and/or weight loss plan. My intention here is to give you some conceptual information that you are probably not aware of and to give you some suggestions of where to begin.

To determine a ball park figure in "how many calories do you need to eat today," we need to account for three aspects: how many calories does your body utilize by just breathing and being alive; for the digestion and elimination of food and all activities that consume calorie expenditures.

- **Resting Metabolism Rate (RMR)** = if you sat in a chair and quietly just read a book with no movement, your RMR is how many calories you would burn. To calculate your RMR refer back to your LBM and multiply that by *10 calories* if you are a woman and *11 calories* if you are a man.

- **Thermic Effects of Food (TEF)** = the amount of energy expenditure that it takes for all of the complex parts of food digestion, assimilation and elimination. (10% of total daily calories for both men and women) To calculate your TEF, multiply your RMR x 10 %.

- **Thermic Effects of Activity (TEA)** = all the other activities that you do in a given day that requires you to burn calories. To calculate your TEA, much like you determined your Protein Prescription earlier, **in the chart below** you need to determine your routine activity level and the corresponding TEA percentage of daily calories.

Add up your RMR and TEF subtotal = _____. Multiply the subtotal number by TEA % in the chart below.

Subtotal _____ x _____TEA% = _____ (TEA) total activity level calories. (see example below)

Physical Activity Level Per Average Day	Thermic Effects of Activity (TEA) % of Daily Calories
Sedentary: no real exercise or activity except activities of daily living	15%

Modestly Active: light yard work, housecleaning, running errands	20%
Moderately Active: leisurely walking, golfing, strenuous yard work	25%
Active Lifestyle: walk/run/cycle at least 3x week for 30 min.	30%
Very Active: Vigorous exercise activity daily for at least 60 min.	35%

- **Total Daily Calories (TDC):** Sum up the RMR + TEF + TEA = TDC.

  Example: Let's take Fred again. If you recall he has an LBM of 150 pounds. To calculate his RMR we multiply 150 x 11 = 1,650. His TEF would be 1,650 x .10 = 165. RMR + TEF (1,650 + 165) = (Subtotal of 1,815.) To calculate TEA%, Fred is moderately active, so we take, 1,815 and multiply x .25 % = 454.

  Fred's TDC = 1650 + 165 + 454 = 2,269 Calories total per day

Total Daily Calories (TDC)

I have given you a formula to calculate a suggested number of calories per day as a *starting place*. This number will vary depending upon your own goals, change in lifestyle habits, and exercise. It is probably accurate within +/- 5 % of the number of calories necessary to keep you at your present weight. One of the key points I want to make, especially for those of you who have done a lot of "yo-yo dieting," going up and down dramatically in caloric intake, is: **never eat fewer calories per day than your Resting Metabolism Rate (RMR).**

The reason is because the RMR is the number of calories that your body needs to maintain its basic metabolic processes. For most individuals, that is going to be at least 1,200 calories for men and 1,000 calories for women, which is about 10–11 calories per pound of LBM. (I tweaked the formula above to accommodate a slight difference between men and women.)

A number of my clients—especially women—believe when I give them this number that it is the maximum **total** number of calories I suggest that they consume. They are shocked when they find out that is the **minimum** number of calories I suggest they eat every day.

The reality is that many women have been eating too few calories. When a person continually eats fewer calories per day than their RMR, the body goes into fasting mode and will begin utilizing protein for fuel. When this happens, you lose muscle mass, which is the biggest calorie burner in your body. And you definitely don't want to do that!

Putting it all together

Your TGPD _____ x 4 calories per gram
=_____ Total Protein Calories Per Day (TPCPD)

Your total TGPD = _____; divide that number by
five = _____Total Grams Protein Per Meal
(TGPM) and insert in the spaces below.

Breakfast _____TGPM

Morning Snack _____TGPM

Lunch _____TGPM

Afternoon Snack _____TGPM

Dinner _____TGPM

All protein sources have 4 calories per gram, so
multiply your TGPM _____ x 4 calories per gram
=_____ your Protein Calories Per Meal
(PCPM).

TDC = _____

- TPCPD = _____

Daily Available
Calories After
Protein (DACAP) = _____
left over to eat low
GI carbs, good fats,
fruit, and dairy
products.

Your DACAP = _____ divided by 5 = _____ Daily Available Calories After Protein Per Meal. (DACAPM)

Week One: This is a trial phase, so you want to carry a notepad with you and jot down ideas and things you want to investigate and perhaps try during weeks two, three, and four. Here are the main points for week one:

1. Start reading all food labels, especially the number of servings per package, serving size, and total calories, as well as the amount of protein, carbohydrates, and fat per serving. Most fast food and quick-serve restaurants now have the Nutrition Information either posted on the wall or in the menu, or they will provide it to you upon request. Vagueness is your worst enemy in this regard.

2. Learn about the Glycemic Index (GI), especially for the foods you routinely eat. Begin eating foods with lower GI values, and be conscious about the higher GI ones that you still choose to eat anyway. My job is to give you the concepts and informational blueprints, and yours is to pick up the tools and utilize them. I do not get into specific recipe and meal planning. From my experience, most books on eating and nutrition quickly get lost into the specific foods themselves, which again takes

the emphasis back to the plate and fork, and not what the food does once it's inside your body.

3. **Eat within 30 minutes of rising in the morning, especially getting your TGPM. This is the most important thing you can do.**

4. Be diligent in getting TGPM every 3 hours, 5 times a day (for example, 6 a.m., 9 a.m., noon, 3 p.m., and 6 p.m.).

5. If you are not sure how many total calories you should shoot for, use the method I supplied as a starting place. I do not suggest that you get obsessive about counting every calorie, but rather have a pretty good idea of how many you are eating in a day. The GBOT is not a weight loss program and is not designed with that purpose in mind, even though a number of you will lose weight/fat during these 4 weeks. Most adults, including nutritionists, constantly underestimate the number of calories they eat and also overestimate their activity levels. Those love handles keep perfect score!

6. I do not suggest a definite hard-and-fast ratio of protein, carbs, and fats such as many new diet/meal planners do. We are trying to get just the right amount of protein, not too much and not too little. Your TPCPD is approximately 20-25% of your TDC, so your DACAP is going to be

a 50/50 split of low GI carbs and good fats spread out evenly over your 3 meals and 2 snacks.

7. Take your DACAP and divide it by 5, and that will give your DACAPM, which is the number of calories to spread out through your 3 meals and 2 snacks. Let your DACAPM be a 50/50 mix (low GI starches and vegetables/good fats) at your 3 meals and 50/50 mix (fruit and dairy/good fats) at your 2 snacks. *Some of you might think this is difficult, eating the same amount of food 5 times a day, meals the same as snacks (I considered calling them all meals, but that would probably confused you more), but the purpose is to stabilize your blood sugar and this is the best way to do it for now.*

8. Make an effort to choose palatable low GI vegetables and/or starches to eat for breakfast, lunch, and dinner.

9. With your mid-morning and afternoon snack, along with your PCPM, eat small portions of either fruit and/or dairy products along with a handful of nuts. It is easy to carry cheese, fruit, or yogurt and a small baggie of nuts with you wherever you go, even if you are on the go all day. Remember to read the labels, because milk products and nuts contain protein, carbs, and fat content in them. If you travel extensively, and the above suggestions are difficult, then you might want to invest in some of the new

nutrition bars such as Balance Bar® or ZonePerfect®. They have a good protein/carb/fat ratio and will do in a pinch.

Here's an example of how to use the numbers. David, a corporate general counsel, has a total of 2,000 TDC, and his TPCPD of protein is 400 calories, so his DACAP is 1,600 left for the day. Using the formula above, 1,600 divided by 5, his DACAPM = 320 calories per 3 meals and 2 snacks, with an equal amount of carbs/fats at meals and snacks. (I told you that you shouldn't be hungry doing this.)

So David's day would look like this:

Each Meal: 80 calories protein, 160 calories low GI carbs, 160 calories good fats. (Remember that carbs have 4 calories per gram and fats have 9 calories per gram.)

Each Snack: 80 calories protein, 160 calories of fruit/dairy product, and 160 calories of good fats.

Your Worksheet

Your TDC =_____calories

Your TPCPD =_____calories

Your DACAP =_____calories

Your DACAP divided by 5 = Your DACAPM_____

Each Meal: PCPM _____
DACAPM_____(50/50 low GI carbs/fats)

Each Snack: PCPM _____
DACAPM_____(50/50 fruit and dairy/fats)

10. For those of you who eat out a lot, this will be a little more difficult, but not overly burdensome. As you know, the "new normal" portion sizes are now much bigger than in the past, and certainly more than most adults (who are not Olympic athletes in training!) should eat at one sitting.

11. For lunch and dinner, order salads, fruit, and/or vegetables a la carte (as side orders), substitutions, or off the menu (just ask, they may likely have it in the kitchen). Breakfast is easier, as restaurants have been offering a la carte items for decades.

12. If you still get the huge "set" meal, here's what I tell my clients: eat half of everything served and you should be good to go. If you are eating meat, roughly the size of a deck of playing

cards is your limit. That is probably about 20 grams of protein, so you've satisfied your TGPM. For the leftovers, ask for a "to go" box if it's possible for you to take it with you (some buffets do not allow this, and even if you can take it, you then have to be able to keep hot food hot and cold food cold for safety). If you can take the other half home, you can eat it tomorrow and get two meals for the price of one!

13. Do not eat anything after 8 p.m.

Week Two: My hope for you after week one of the GBOT Program is that your carb cravings are under control, you have more energy, and your blood sugar is more stable. If you have succeeded in doing this, you are well on your way! Here are suggestions to consider during week two:

1. For those of you who are *still* craving carbs, let me ask, have you been diligently eating your prescribed amount of protein every 3 hours and 5 separate, evenly-spaced meals/snacks? If not, then repeat week one, following the suggested program exactly.

2. If you have followed the suggestions for week one to the letter and you are *still* experiencing the cravings, try this. If your TGPD was 60 grams; add an additional 50% for the second week. That would be 60 x 0.5 = 30 additional

grams of protein daily (now 90 grams), or going from about 12 grams per meal up to 18 grams per meal/snack. Just add the extra calories to your regimen and press on. If you do this for the second week, there is a great likelihood that the carb cravings will go away this week. Keep eating the same number of calories and 50/50 carb/fat ratio at each meal/snack as in week one.

3. If you were experiencing carb cravings before week one, and they now have **diminished**, then the protein is working as it should, so don't make any changes to your protein prescription. This week you should feel even better and have more clarity and energy. However, let's tweak your DACAPM to focus on eating a little more low GI carbs and a little less good fats. Take the 50/50 ratio that we used in week one and change it to 60% low GI carbs and 40% good fats. So your new ratio will be 60/40 for your DACAPM. Keep eating the same number of calories at each meal/snack as in week one.

Week Three: If you have been diligent both weeks with the protein prescription/eating plan *to the letter*, your real carb cravings should be gone. I cannot recall any client I have ever worked with who followed my suggestions whose cravings did *not* subside within two weeks. You should now have more energy and better mental acuity as a result of learning how to use food to your maximum advantage. Here are some additional suggestions for week three.

1. For those of you who were *not* diligent in following the suggestions for the first week but *did* follow the entire program for week two, your carb cravings should be vanquished or greatly reduced. In either case, since you are a little behind the rest of the class so to speak, you will have to play catch-up. So for week three, go back to **week two** above and follow the plan in # 2.

2. For those of you, who were still craving carbs in week two and added 50% more protein to your new TGPD, stay at that level for now. I want you to get the ongoing experience of not having carb cravings, and see that you *do* have the power of control over sugar; that by simply learning not only what to eat, but when and how much, can make all the difference in the world. Until you get the carb cravings under control, it's almost impossible to work on weight loss or other nutritional goals.

   As we did for the other group last week, let's tweak your DACAPM to focus on eating a little more low GI carbs and a little less good fats. Take the 50/50 ratio that we used in week one and change it to 60% low GI carbs and 40% good fats. So your new ratio will be 60/40 for your DACAPM. Keep eating the same number of calories at each meal/snack.

3. For those who were *not* experiencing any carb cravings in week two, keep up the good work. Since you now know that the targeted protein/eating plan has helped you with your hormonal balance, instead of dividing your TGPD by 5 equal amounts, let's take part of the morning and afternoon snacks and put them back into your 3 normal meals. Take the 40% of your TGPD that you were using toward both of your snacks and cut that amount by half, down to 20%, and then spread that extra 20% evenly on breakfast and lunch.

For example: If your TGPD is 100 grams x 0.40 = 40 grams (TGPM is 20 grams in the morning snack and TGPM is also 20 grams for the afternoon snack). Cut each snack back to 10 grams and add 10 grams to breakfast and lunch. So now your 100 TGPD would be: 30 TGPM for breakfast and 30 TGPM lunch, 20 TGPM for dinner, and 10 TGPM for morning and afternoon snacks.

Also, and instead of dividing your DACAP by 5, let's spread out your DACAPM snack calories. Take the DACAPM at both snacks, and cut that amount by half, and spread it evenly at breakfast and lunch, still using the same 60/40 carb/fat ratio.

For example: If your DACAP = 1,600 calories (your DACAPM was 320 calories for each meal and snack), now take 320 and divide by 2 = 160 calories. Your new DACAPM for breakfast and lunch is 320 + 160 = 480 calories. Dinner would remain the same as the original DACAPM of 320 calories. So your new DACAPM would be:

o Breakfast = 480 calories (60/40 carb/fat)

o Morning Snack = 160 calories (60/40 carb fat)

o Lunch = 480 calories (60/40 carb fat)

o Afternoon Snack = 160 calories (60/40 carb/fat)

o Dinner = 320 calories (60/40 carb/fat)

Week Four: Alright boys and girls, gather around the campfire! If you have been diligent in following my suggestions, you have made great progress. Just as the Get-Back-On-Track name implies, I have helped you make a beginning, and given you some information that you can use for the rest of your life, wherever you go. Remember, fundamentals (like blocking and tackling in football) are the key. Now that your body is responding, the work left has to do with your mind. I am reminded of that great Vince Lombardi quote, "The good Lord gave you a body that can stand most anything. It's your mind you have to convince." Here are some suggestions for week four:

1. For those you playing catch-up last week, go back to week three and follow the plan in suggestion #2. To use a medical analogy, if you had a bacterial strep throat infection and went to your doctor, she would want to not only determine the right medication, but also the right dosage and length of time to stay on it to make sure you kill the bug. It's always better to do a little too much to make sure you kill the bug than do it incorrectly, and have the bug come back stronger than ever. In the same way, we want to make sure that you get your carb cravings under control, so stay with this plan for the fourth week.

2. For those of you who added the extra 50% of protein to your new and higher TGPD, how is that working? If it's working and ALL of your carb cravings have disappeared, cut back the amount of extra protein by one-half. In other words, cut back one-half of the extra 50% to your original TGPD + 25%. Try this and see how it works. You might have to play with the protein prescription to find out what works for you. With your new slightly-lower TGPD, go back to week three and follow the revised eating plan in #3.

3. For the other group of you who had great success in the first week and your crab cravings

went away, continue following week three #3. If it worked well, then stay with what works.

Information for all groups

4. Educate yourself about a newer concept called the *Glycemic Load (GL)*, which is a much more sophisticated measure than the Glycemic Index. The GI only tells you **how fast** a carbohydrate turns into sugar, but the GL tells you **how much** of that carbohydrate is in a serving of a specific food. This takes into account the amount of fiber and water that I mentioned earlier. For instance, carrots have a surprisingly high GI but a moderate GL, due to their high fiber and water content, which allows for only a small amount of active carbohydrate per serving that one assimilates. In other words, you would have to eat a pound of carrots to have a real effect on blood sugar.

    Most foods that have a low GI will also have a corresponding low GL, but there are some carbs with a surprisingly high GI that have a *low* GL. If this is too much detail, that's fine; staying with the knowledge of GI alone is a good way to live. I just wanted to impart this information for those of you who want to refine your food choices.

5. Are you staying hydrated? Probably not yet. Most of my female clients are dehydrated, especially in the warm months here in the Deep

South. Back to my fundamental principle, how much liquid (water) should you drink? Probably more! With all of today's palatable beverage choices that have little or no calories, including all of the new flavored water drinks, you should be able to drink more. Remember, if you are thirsty, you are already behind the curve. Also, drink a beverage 10 minutes before you eat a meal; it will help you feel fuller.

6. Are you eating enough fiber? Again, the answer is probably *no*. If you concentrate on eating MORE veggies, and a small amount of fruit (we discussed why you don't want to eat fruit in abundance if you want to lose weight), it will help. Once the Captain of an ocean liner gives the command to turn the ship, it might take up to 7 miles to complete the task. So, keep at it. If you have specific questions, ask your doctor.

7. Stay away from all of the late-night infomercials about this type of diet or that. The basic principles of human physiology and carbohydrate and protein metabolism have not changed recently. I am often amused when a client asks me about some new "berry" that they read about on the Internet that promises this or that health benefit, when the client is 50 pounds overweight and can't walk around the block. First things first!

Going forward

Depending upon how diligent you followed the plan and how you responded during the four weeks, by now your carb cravings should be under control. If you have mastered this, you should have the confidence and motivation to take on whatever other nutritional and/or weight loss goals that you want to going forward. Experiment with your calorie intake and find the best level that works for you. It will change as your goals change, so keep that in mind. The plan that was laid out in week three #3 is what I would recommend if your goal is maintenance.

Exercise

On the move

The human body was meant to move–and when we move we use our muscles. That IS the issue. We don't move enough and we don't use our muscles. For most of us, our *new normal* is that we sit at a desk all day and then get into our car and drive home and sit on the couch until we go to bed at night and eating all the time without little or no real movement or exertion on our parts. Even though this is normal, it is NOT natural.

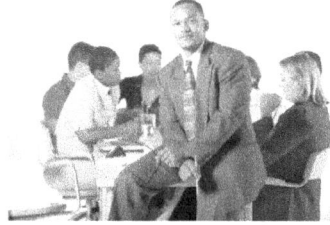

Based on my experience as a personal trainer and working with hundreds of clients, my exercise suggestions below are designed to help lower your blood glucose levels, increase your energy and stamina and to assist you to begin exercising again or maybe this is the very first time. The strength training is designed to be a refresher course for people who have done resistance/weight training in the past or a great beginner program for those of you who might have never exercised.

Check with your physician

Before you begin participating in any exercise program, including this one, please check with your physician or qualified health provider to determine if it is safe to proceed. The author specifically disclaims any liability, loss, or risk that is incurred as a consequence.

Movement

Besides the many positive benefits of regular exercise, when we move the body, all of our muscle cells utilize the glucose already available in the cell and then after this is depleted, the cells pull glucose out of the bloodstream which in turn lowers blood glucose levels.

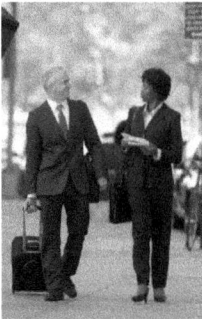

Also, movement will help insulin become more efficient at transporting glucose into the cells more rapidly, which again naturally lowers blood glucose levels.

Here is my suggestion for everyone during all four weeks:

Just as I have advised you to eat 5-times a day to help better balance blood sugar, let's utilize your valuable time by using walking to maximum effect on stabilizing your blood sugar levels. If possible, wait 45-60 minutes after you eat every meal/snack and then get up and take a walk for 5-minutes. The 45-60 minutes after you eat is the approximate time that most of your blood sugar levels will peak while eating a low GI carb diet and the 5-minute walk will help to bring down your blood glucose levels in the ways that I have described. Go at whatever pace feels comfortable, and if you can't do it for all 5 meals/snacks, then do what you can. It all adds up and will benefit you.

Walking machine

The body can run, but it's the most amazing walking machine ever devised. Unlike our distant ancestors who walked on all fours, we humans have perfect balance and can use our hands to accomplish any task that we want to perform. Also, we have built-in closet space for an almost unlimited storage supply of energy: fat.

Accumulating fat was supposed to be our insurance policy against starvation; like a business line of credit from the bank you can draw on when you have a cash flow crunch due to the fluctuations in the business cycle. Instead, it has literally become the millstone around our neck.

When clients ask me how much they should walk, my general response again, is **MORE**, *up to the point of your physical limit or medical condition.* It doesn't matter for how long, how slow/fast you walk, just walk, because your primary goal is to assist your body to overcome the carb cravings.

In addition to the benefits described above, movement triggers the Pancreas to secrete the fasting hormone Glucagon, which naturally raises your blood sugar level and mobilizes your body to begin burning fat for fuel.

Strengthen your muscles

Besides increasing our strength and making our muscle mass grow, adding more metabolically active muscle uses more glucose which helps to lower blood glucose levels, as well.

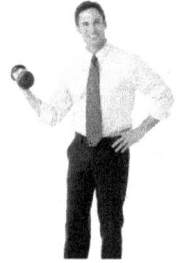

We will focus on exercising our upper bodies. It is the most efficient use of your time since your legs are generally stronger than your upper body if you have been sedentary, especially if you are carrying extra weight. In that case, every step you take has been a lower body exercise. I think you get the picture. I will show you how to perform each exercise below.

Each exercise demonstration is called one *repetition* (rep). Ten repetitions equal one *set*. So if I suggest that you do 2 sets of the exercise daily that means performing 10 reps, take a one minute break, and then perform the second set, for a total of 20 reps.

Basic exercises

Abdominals: (Abs) You do not need to do elaborate crunches like you see the young guys doing in the gym to develop strong abs. Since all a muscle can do is contract, however you can isolate it and put the muscle into overload, it will respond. This exercise strengthens your *rectus abdominis* and *transverse rectus abdominis* muscles. I am going to demonstrate for you 2 different ways that you can perform these.

Chair: Find a comfortable chair with a straight back, like an informal chair at the kitchen table. As you can see on the **left,** I am slouching with my legs crossed and both feet on the floor with my hands folded and my back straight. Poke one hand 2-inches above your naval and push in hard. Lift your crossed feet 2-4 inches, as you see on the **right,** very slowly, and hold for 2-4 seconds. Very slowly, return your feet to the floor. Did you feel your muscles contracting? If so, you just did an effective exercise that is comparable to a crunch. This is one repetition.

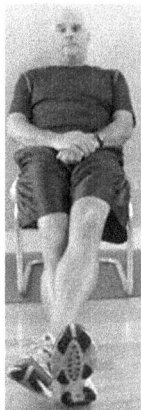

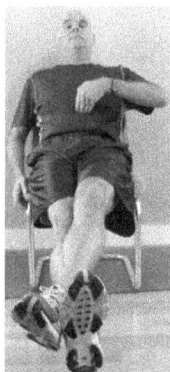

Floor: If you find it more comfortable to do your ab work on the floor, here is another demonstration of it being done. Lay on the floor, as you see on the **left,** cross your feet, place both of your hands behind your head interlocking your fingers to supply support for your neck. Very slowly, lift your crossed feet 2-4 inch up as you see **above,** and hold the

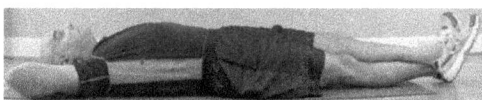

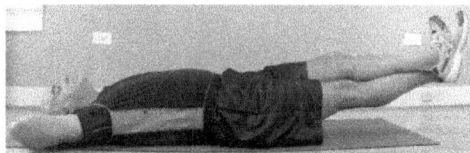

position for 2-4 seconds. Very slowly, return your feet to the floor. This is one repetition.

Exercise Suggestions: Choose one of the methods above to perform the ab exercise. Week One: 1 set daily. Week Two: 2 sets daily. Week Three: 3 sets daily. Week Four: 3 sets daily.

Side Abdominals: If you put your hand down on the sides of your stomach about half way between your belly button and your side you will feel another set of muscles called our *internal* and *external obliques.* They are sometimes referred to as our love handles. We use these muscles to help us turn and for many other useful functions. Lay on the ground and curl your legs and knees and put your head under your head to support your neck. Put your hand in the middle of the position between your navel and side as you see to the **left.** Very slowly lift your crossed feet together about 2-4 inches as you see to the **right**. You should feel your muscles contracting there as well. Hold for 2-4 seconds, and then very slowly return your feet to the floor. Now, turn over on your other side and repeat the same process. Completing both sides is one repetition.

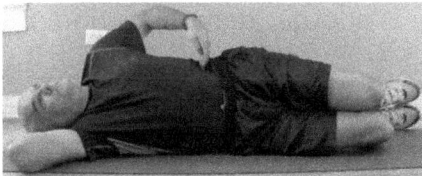

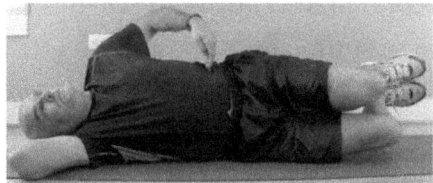

Exercise Recommendations: Week One: 1 set daily. Week Two: 2 sets daily. Week Three: 3 sets daily. Week Four: 3 sets daily.

<u>Pushups</u>: This exercise is the single best overall exercise you can do for your upper body. Unlike the full pushups that most of us are familiar with, below are two variations that don't strain your back and you still benefit.

Wall pushups: These are great and anyone can do them whatever your fitness or strength level is. All you need is a good bare wall. Stand in front of a wall, feet about shoulder width apart, arms stretched out with palms on the wall about 6 inches below your shoulders as you see on the **left**. Now slowly lower yourself to the wall keeping your elbows tucked in tight and your back straight till your nose touches the wall for 2-4 seconds as you see on the **right.** Push yourself back up to the starting position. This is one repetition.

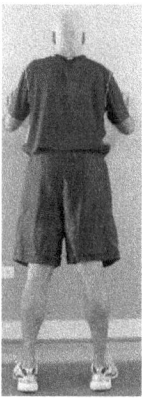

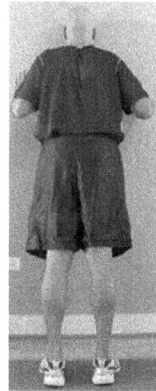

Note: You can experiment with different feet and hand positions. As you move your feet away from the wall, the pushups become progressively harder. You may need to lower your hand position on the wall.

Floor ½ pushups: Lay down on the floor on your stomach in the regular pushup position, elbows in tight. Cross your legs and lift your feet up perpendicular to the floor as you see here on the **left.** Now slowly push yourself straight up using your arms and shoulders, keeping your elbows tight against your body and your back straight for 2-4 seconds as you see on the **right.** Lower yourself back to the ground in the starting position. This is one repetition.

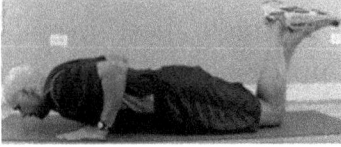

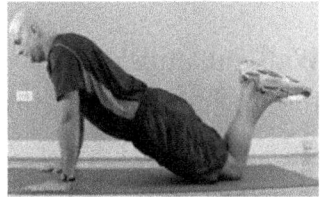

Exercise Recommendations: Choose one of the methods above to perform the pushups. Week One: 1 set daily. Week Two: 2 sets daily. Week Three: 2 sets daily. Week Four: 2 sets daily.

Dumbbells and resistance tubes

I am demonstrating the following exercises using dumbbells and resistance tubes, which are similar to the flat bands, but the tubes have handles and last longer. Generally, the darker the color of the resistance tube, the higher the resistance. They go from black to bright yellow and can be found along with dumbbells in most sports stores. I have used both dumbbells and tubes with my clients and so go with your own preference.

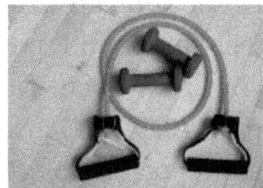

Choosing the right starting weight or resistance level is easy. Go to the sports store and pick up the dumbbells or resistance tubes and choose the one that you can perform somewhere *between* 5-10 reps of the bicep curl (see pg. 63). That is your good beginning weight. One advantage of using the tubes is that by moving your hands down from the handles and choking up on the tubes, you increase the resistance.

As you go through the four weeks and you get stronger, you will probably have to invest in an additional set of dumbbells or the next level of resistance tube. That is proof that you are getting stronger.

Chest Press: (Resistance tube) Sit up straight with the tube placed behind the back of the chair, firmly

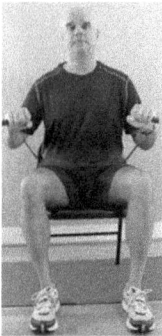

holding the tube handles with palms facing *down* about mid-chest high as see on the **left**. *Remember you can choke up on the tube to increase the resistance.* Keep your elbows tucked in tight and slowly push straight forward with both arms extended and touch

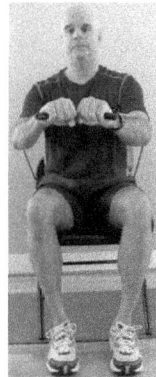

your fists together as you see on the **right,** hold for 2-4 seconds and then return your arms back to the original position. This is one repetition.

(Be careful that the tube doesn't slip up over the top of the chair and hit you in the back).

(Dumbbells) Lay on your back on the floor with feet tucked and your knees high and elbows touching the floor with dumbbells in both hands palms facing *down* as you see on the **left.** Slowly raise and extend both arms and hold for 2-4 seconds as you see on the **right.** Then return your elbows to the floor. This is one repetition.

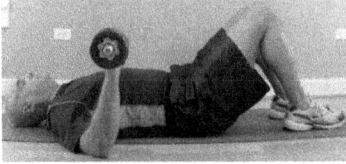

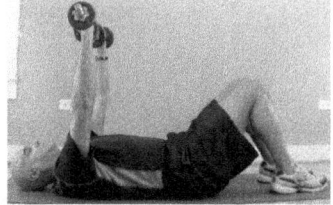

Exercise Recommendations: Choose one of the methods above to perform the chest press. Week One: 1 set daily. Week Two: 1 set daily. Week Three: 2 sets daily. Week Four: 2 sets daily.

Pectoral Muscles: (Resistance tube) Sit up straight with the tube placed behind the back of the chair, firmly holding the tube handles with palms facing *inward* about mid-chest high as see on the **left.** Keep your elbows tucked in tight and slowly push straight forward with both arms extended and then touch your fists together and you should feel your pectorals (chest muscles) tighten as you see on the **right,** hold for 2-4 seconds and then return your arms

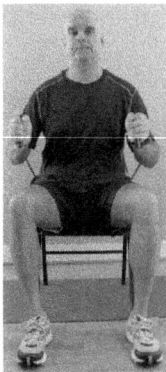

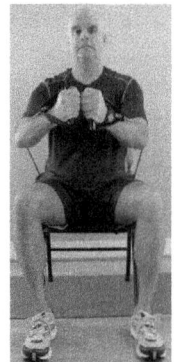

back to the original position. This is one repetition.

(Dumbbells) Lay on your back with feet tucked, knees high and elbows touching the floor with dumbbells in both hands palms facing *inward* as you see on the **left.** Slowly raise and fully extend both arms touching the dumbbells together, you should feel your pectorals (chest muscles) tighten as you see on the **right,** and hold for 2-4 seconds. Then return your elbows to the floor. This is one repetition.

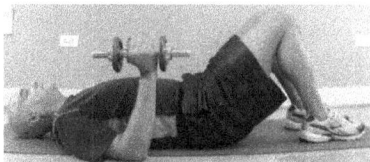

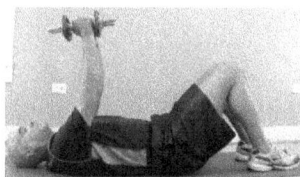

Exercise Recommendations: Choose one of the methods above to perform the pectoral muscle routine. Week One: 1 set daily. Week Two: 1 set daily. Week Three: 2 sets daily. Week Four: 2 sets daily

Bicep Curls: (Resistance tube) Sit up straight with your feet spread apart about shoulder width. Put the tube under your feet holding the handles with your palms facing *upward* and your elbows anchored against your body as you see on the **left.** Keep your weight on the tube with your heels as this is anchoring the resistance.

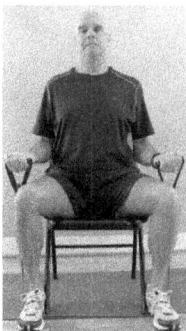

Slowly lift your right arm up to shoulder height as you see on the **right**. You should feel your bicep muscle working. Hold for 2-4 seconds and then slowly return to the starting position. Now repeat the process with your left arm. Completing both sides is one repetition.

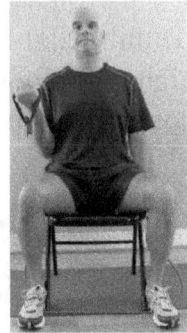

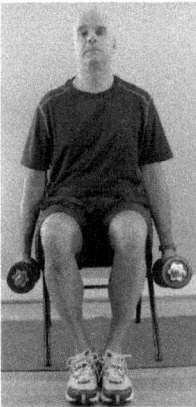

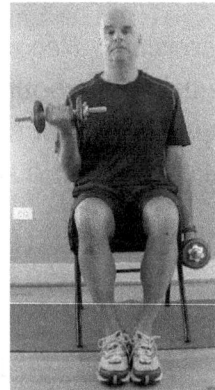

(Dumbbells) Sit up straight in the chair, hold dumbbells in each hand at your side with your palms facing *inward* as you on the **left**. Slowly lift your right arm, and when it is perpendicular with the ground, turn your wrist outward, so that as you see on the **right**, your palm is now facing *upward* and continue lifting your arm to shoulder height as you see on the right. You should feel your bicep muscle working. Hold for 2-4 seconds and then slowly return to the starting position. Now repeat the process with your left arm. Completing both sides is one repetition.

Exercise Recommendations: Choose one of the methods above to perform the bicep curls. Week One: 1 set daily. Week Two: 2 sets daily. Week Three: 3 sets daily. Week Four: 4 sets daily.

Tricep Kickbacks: (Resistance tube not using handles) Sit up straight in the chair hold the tube with your left hand as you see on the **left** and grasp the tube with your right hand about 18-24 inches away from your left hand. Make sure that you keep both elbows tightly pressed against your body. Now fully extend your right arm keeping it against your side and lock your elbow. Hold for 2-4 seconds as you see on the **right**. You will feel your tricep muscle engaging. Slowly return your arm to the starting position keeping it tucked in tight against the body. Now repeat the process with your left arm. Completing both sides is one repetition.

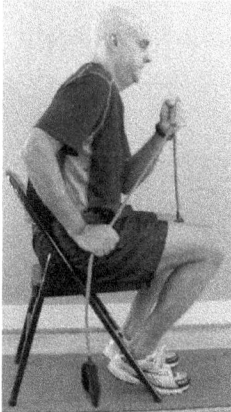

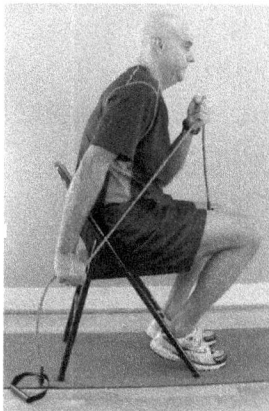

(Dumbbells) Sit in the chair leaning forward about 30 degrees. Hold one dumbbell in your right hand with your palm facing *inward* and your arm straight down and pressed closely against your side as you see on the **left**. Now fully extend your right arm keeping it against your side and lock your elbow. You might find yourself leaning forward up to 45 degrees as you extend your arm, that's ok. Hold for 2-4 seconds as you see on the **right**. You will feel your tricep muscle engaging. Slowly return your arm to the starting position keeping it tucked in tight against the body. Now repeat the process with your left arm. Completing both sides is one repetition.

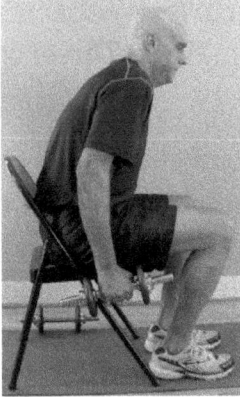

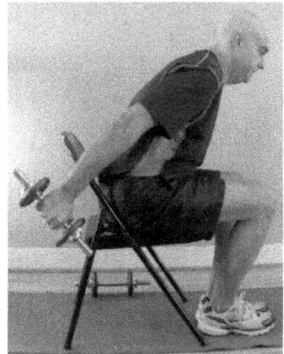

Exercise Recommendations: Choose one of the methods above to perform the tricep kickbacks. Week One: 1 set daily. Week Two: 2 sets daily. Week Three: 3 sets daily. Week Four: 4 sets daily.

Conclusion

Congratulations! You should now have control over your carb cravings, have a good foundation on how to eat and be headed toward getting moderately aerobically fit and significantly stronger. And, you have gotten back-on-track in reclaiming your most valuable asset–you!

Your job now is to stay-on-track. Seek out new information, set goals for yourself and good luck to all of you!

www.ingramcontent.com/pod-product-compliance
Lightning Source LLC
Chambersburg PA
CBHW060634280326
41933CB00012B/2032